Sentiments of

Melody J. Cole

Sentiments of a Survivor

Self-published by Melody J. Cole using KDP

Nonfiction

Cover Design: Graphic designer Shane Cole
Author photographer: Ross W. Cole – edited by Roma Kerns
Editor: Anna Rhea

ISBN: 978-1-7349342-0-5

Dear team,

This book is dedicated to *you!*

God the Father, God the Son, and *God the Holy Spirit* - thank You first and foremost that I have already beaten cancer once! Thank You for helping me write this book. Thank You for the rest of my teams. Thank You for being my Lord, my Savior and my Stylist!

My family - thank you to my paternal grandparents, Ralph and Dorothy; my maternal grandparents, Roy and Marjorie; my parents, Ross and Lois; my brother Shane; my aunts, Roma and Bonnie; my mom's cousin Teresa, my cousin Jenni and her daughter Kylie, and the rest of my family. I am thankful for the roles you play in my life. Thank you to Dad, Shane and Aunt Roma for also helping me with my book cover and author photograph.

My "cancer family" who have gone through cancer personally - thank you to Brandon and Terrah; Krista, my cancer support group and others who supported me through my journey, even as you struggled through your own! You inspired me by sharing your stories and letting me share mine with you.

My medical team - thank you to Scott, Carolyn and others who helped me through treatment. No matter what type of medical capacity you treated me in...whether we agreed or not...you influenced my journey. I thank all of you for helping me get to this side of cancer. Thank you to those who are treating who I am *after* cancer.

My friends - thank you to Tracy, Marcus and Tristian; Rachael, Stephanie, Sheila, Kate, Ron, Doug, Mary, Hensley, and many others for showing me what true friendship is in the face of this adversity I call life! I thank you for listening to me through my cancer journey and beyond. Thank you to those who helped me to and through months of appointments and for your aftercare. I value every friendship!

My book team - to Anna my editor, thank you for helping me make my two-dimensional story that I thought made perfect sense, a clearer three-dimensional story. To my friends and endorsers - Meggie, David, Mark, and Melanie, thank you for being there to help me with my perspective by sharing yours. Thank you to my "writing partner" Earl of Whiskers for sticking close to me while I type this story, whether reminding me to stay on task or take a break.

Those who shall remain nameless - thank you for making a big impact on my little story no matter which team you are on.

Life is beautiful,

Melody J. Cole

Introduction

"Make your mess your message."
- Robin Roberts, news anchor on Good Morning America

  I decided the best way to inform Aunt Roma of my cancer diagnosis was to write her a letter and give her as many details as I thought she would want. Her mom, my Grandma Dorothy, died of ovarian cancer when I was fifteen years old so that had to be part of the details in the letter. You'll understand *why* later.

  After receiving that letter, she sent a care package to me. That package included two journals: one that was hot pink and one with pretty flowers on the cover. In the hot pink journal, I wrote about some of my fears and frustrations and the faith, family, friends, and fun that helped me get to the other side of cancer. Mom told me that I should write a journal that "others could read." She then exclaimed, "You're such a good writer!"

  Oftentimes, I receive information and feel as though I must *do* something with it instead of just *holding* it in my brain. My cancer journey was one of those times. I knew I wasn't going to be able to fight this battle and just forget about it, so the journal with the pretty flowers on the cover became the one that "others could read."

It is designed to be read as it was written. Sometimes I was able to write about a few days at a time, and sometimes I had to write about one day at a time and just say, "Okay, that's enough." This is a true story with a prayer at the end of each day. Read it all at once if you wish. If it is too emotionally charged for you, read it one day at a time. Read it at your own pace.

I began writing this book on July 2, 2016. I was celebrating my first anniversary as a breast cancer survivor. God gave me this story to tell. However, there were several circumstances that I let stop me from telling it for a period of time. As I like to say, "Life gets in the way of life sometimes." Sometimes other people have told my story without my permission. This made me stop telling it when I should have told more of it instead. Sometimes I found myself nervous about sharing my story with people who were affected by cancer in a more gut-wrenching way than I. I told myself that they didn't want to hear my story because they had their own. I quickly lost that thought, after realizing that I was seeing those people like big, mean, ugly ogres just because I feared telling them my story. When I think about this preconceived notion, two men in particular come to mind. Neither one is, nor ever was, such an ogre. In fact, each of them *asked* to hear my story after they heard *about* it! That makes proclaiming it now much easier than it used to be. By the way, neither one of them is ugly!

I've heard it said that you should never be ashamed of *your story*...because it's *your story* and there is no wrong way to tell it, if *you* are the one telling the story. I think I am ready to continue the tale.

On my Survivor Day in 2019, I decided it was time to finish writing this book and I set a deadline for myself to finally be self-published by July 2, 2020 – my fifth anniversary of being a cancer survivor. I celebrate being a survivor on July 2nd because I received the results of the first clear mammogram on that day in 2015. I call it my Survivor Day because of something Mom said the morning of July 2, 2017. She was spending the weekend with me to help celebrate. She woke me in the morning, giving me a kiss on the cheek with a big smile on her face, and said, "Happy Survivor Day!" Unfortunately, that was the last Survivor Day I would spend with her here on Earth. Her own battle with cancer began later that same year. But, that's another book for another time.

Hopefully, if you are reading this right now, that means that I set my goal on time, or maybe even a little early! I encourage you to read it, enjoy it, and start working towards setting one of *your* goals today! This book is in no way, shape or form supposed to be an exact "how-to" guide for surviving cancer. It is the way I am making my "mess" my "message." I realize that many do not go through cancer treatment as easily as I did...and many do not make it through their earthly battle with cancer. Right now, I do not have words to adequately describe how hard that must be or how hard it is to watch a loved one suffer through it.

Originally, I thought this book was going to be about my journey through cancer. I have since realized that, although I am a survivor, the journey continues and always will. I hope to be able to continue the checkups, the testing, and meeting wonderful people who have been through something similar. This is merely a short summary of my own journey of coming through to the other side of cancer while here on Earth.

I pray that it inspires you, makes you laugh, think, and gives you the courage to fight your own battle. Each of us in this fight is as individual as the diagnosis, treatment and outcome of this thing we call, *"the big c."* So, whether you are currently battling *the big c* or have in the past, I hope this book helps you.

Most, if not all of us, know someone affected by cancer. If that is the case, please read this book so you might gain a better understanding of what they may be going through...and then give one to them. I would love for this book to end up in cancer treatment centers across the nation! I feel as though it is my duty to use the gifts God gave me, so I pray that these words help at least one person.

The Big C

On the evening of June 23, 2014, I was lying in bed when I felt a terrible itch on my right breast. Yes, I said *itch*. Now, there will be a few moments while reading this book in which you might say, "Melody! TMI!" Here is the first...but probably not the last. When I was younger, I would feel an itch on the right side of my chest whenever I was around a cute boy, kind of like a nervous itch. As I got older this itch persisted whenever I saw an attractive male. As I have gotten older still the nervous itch has not come to me nearly as often as it used to...no offense to any handsome gentlemen! I'd like to think as I've matured, my taste in men has as well! Anyway, I digress. Point is, at that particular moment I was alone and knew without a doubt that that itch was *not* a nervous reaction.

I am blessed to feel very little pain or discomfort in my lower body because I was born partially paralyzed due to spina bifida - a condition that occurs when at least two vertebrae of the spine are misaligned. So, when I do feel discomfort from something as simple as an itch, it is intensified and really hurts! I figured the itch in question was simply a bug bite...and fell asleep. Yet, the next morning I discovered that there was no bug bite. As I felt around the spot where the itch had been the night before, I felt a lump instead.

I knew how to do a self-breast exam but had never gotten into a good routine of doing one. I discussed this during the initial appointment with my new doctor, and she agreed that we could discuss breast exams during my next visit, and she would remind me how to do one. Unfortunately, I felt this itch in between appointments so our talk about exams came after my diagnosis.

Other issues, such as fragile lower extremities that break easier than they bend, and severe reactions to any medication that enters my bloodstream too rapidly, made treatment a unique and trying experience for me...and that's putting it mildly! I will discuss reasons for the uniqueness later.

I felt blessed to feel the spot and lump, especially since I did not have a good routine of self-examination at the time. I was also blessed to have a medical appointment for wound care treatment with a nurse practitioner – a former oncology nurse – already scheduled at the hospital for the next day.

Physically, the only two options I have are sitting in my wheelchair or lying down all day. Throughout my life I have had periods of time of treatment by wound care specialists for pressure sores. Sometimes these periods are quite long. I had been seeing this specialist for about six months, so I was extremely comfortable around her. I let her feel

the lump, and she confirmed my suspicion that I
needed to get it checked out. The nurse practitioner
contacted my primary care doctor for me, and
within a week, at the age of thirty-five, I had my
first two mammograms, and a biopsy. On July 2,
2014, my doctor called me herself to give me the
shocking news.

I had breast cancer!

The last statistic that I heard was that 80% of
breast cancers are *not* hereditary. Although many
members of my family have had cancer, I am the
first one to have had breast cancer. As far as I know
I am still the only one in my family who has had it
and for that, I am *glad*! I rarely go through a "Why
me?" phase. Having breast cancer was no different.
Instead I kept thinking "Why *not* me?"

Cancer is not something I would wish on my
own worst enemy. I'm glad I had it. Yes, I said it,
I'm *glad*! I am so used to being a patient that I
worry more about how my illness is going to affect
others. I *know* how I am going to get through it. A
few years after I had cancer, I watched Mom struggle
with her cancer and that was much harder, especially
since her struggle ended in death.

Grandma Marjorie struggled with
Alzheimer's Disease for the last four or five years of
her life. Mom and several others in our family took
turns helping Grandpa take care of her twenty-four
hours a day, seven days a week after a bad fall she
had which resulted in her breaking her leg. She had

more than her fair share of illnesses (i.e., two unexplained seizures, pneumonia at least twice) during that time, but she never had cancer. I remember commenting to Mom during my first chemotherapy treatment that I'm glad we didn't have to go through this with Grandma because it would have complicated the situation. She agreed.

In some cases, breast cancer can be genetically linked to ovarian cancer in another family member. Grandma Dorothy had had ovarian cancer, so my oncologist ordered a blood test to determine if our cancers could be connected. After further testing and a few frequently exhausting medical appointments, it was discovered that our cancers were not connected.

I found out I had Stage 1A, Grade 3, Triple Negative, Invasive Mammary Carcinoma with medullary features with the possibility of aggressive growth, A.K.A., breast cancer that *was not* linked to Grandma's ovarian cancer...in my right breast. Wow! That's a mouthful for such a small lump! I have received many diagnoses in my lifetime (literally from head to toe) but the "and now this!" feeling I had when diagnosed with cancer came with the realization that this one was going to change my life forever.

Lord, I pray for my readers who are anticipating or have just gotten a diagnosis of "The Big C!" Please let them know that it does not have to be so scary when You are on the journey with them. Amen

~~~

Day 2

I'm too young!

I was only thirty-five years old when I had my first mammogram. Leading radiologists suggest that women begin to have yearly mammograms at the age of forty. Many would say that age thirty-five is too young for an initial mammogram. I was told that my doctor might not suggest a mammogram, even though I found a lump, just because I was so young. I agree! It should be too young to *have* to have your first mammogram. However, it is *never* too early to learn what your body is supposed to feel like. It is *never* too early to consult a doctor if something feels abnormal.

While I was being prepped for a needle localization (a procedure that preceded my lumpectomy) Carolyn, the operating room nurse said that the hospital had recently seen a surge of women with breast cancer that were in their early thirties. And I thought *I* was too young! Maybe thirty-five is not too early for an initial mammogram after all?

Every good mammogram result (I frame mine!) comes with the strong suggestion to start regular mammograms at the age of forty. I chuckle every time I see that. It's not "ha-ha" funny, but it surprises me that forty is still considered the right age for regular exams. Breast cancer can occur so much earlier in life! By the way, I put all my good mammogram results in a frame behind a puzzle of an hourglass. The hourglass reminds me of the last image taken during the first clear mammogram I had. Need I say more?

I believe God gave me the itch, literally, so I would get the spot checked. I was already under the care of a nurse practitioner and a surgeon who were in regular contact with my primary physician. That was such a blessing! Cancer breaks down a person's immune system and can slow healing, so that may have had something to do with the trouble with my skin at the time. To this day I wonder which came first, the chicken or the egg? If a person's skin is fragile and he/she has a skin breakdown while having cancer it can take up to six years for the skin to heal, which might look different than it did before they had cancer.

I don't say that to scare anyone or gain sympathy. I have been advised more than once to be detailed about certain aspects of my life in order to illicit a better understanding of my story, so I am doing so.

I had to resume wound care treatment after I left my most recent job (more about that later), and I still receive it. I have gone through long stretches of time when treatment has really helped, and then times when I slack on my part of the healing process and go the other direction. Right now, I'd say I'm doing well!

When I moved away to college, I had to start taking care of the logistics of my medical care on my own. Mom was always what I would call "fussy" when it came to what I needed, especially pertaining to my medical care. She was persnickety about the way I was treated and was never shy about speaking up for me. I started to appreciate and imitate that attitude more than ever when dealing with medical issues on my own. Dad has the same attitude, but he has also had to remind me to "Be nice!" I have learned to ask a lot of questions until I get the answers I need.

I must depend on the competence of caretakers and other medical professionals to let me know if they see something abnormal that I may not be able to see or feel. It is such a blessing to have others helping me take care of my body when I have competent people to help me! On the other hand, I've had medical professionals who do not know how to properly treat my body. I know all of us make mistakes...but...*that sucks*!

I turned forty-years-old in 2018 and I have already had more than my fair share of mammograms in the last five years. I guess if I *had* to have cancer, I can at least be thankful that I am able to have those tests that let me know whether I still have ned (no evidence of disease). I can already say that I have *beaten* breast cancer once and that is a bit of a relief since I know the alternative. For that, I am extremely thankful!

God, if there are men or women reading this in fear of getting an abnormality tested, please take away that fear and help them find the right answers. Amen.

~~~

Day 3

"The only thing we have to fear is fear itself."
Former President Franklin Delano Roosevelt in his
first Inaugural speech

Before I was diagnosed with cancer, I went through a time when I was fearful about many things. Some of the fear stemmed from not feeling safe around someone I worked with closely. She had someone in her life who was not safe for her to be around. I feared for her all the time, and sometimes I feared for myself when I was around her, although I had never met her abuser. Some other people in my life were also concerned for my safety. Eventually, I realized that, as long as I was appropriately cautious, fear for myself was unnecessary. I continuously prayed for *her* safety.

Usually, when I decide I want something, I go for it before spending much time on thinking about how I will go for it. I find that if I spend too much time planning, I will find a reason that I *can't do* something, and I quit the pursuit. This goes against everything I believe! I am content with the way my life is going, most of the time. But, I suppose that most of us, if honest, wish we were older, younger, more professional, more successful...overall at a different place in life at times. I am no different, and this was one of those times for me. Once I really took time to honestly think about it, I thought to myself, "How am I *ever* going to *get* where I want to be in life?" For example, God willing, one day I will become a wife and another day I will become a mom. For some reason, this fearful time in my life came with the uncertainty of being able to fulfill these dreams.

I had a lot of time to dwell on this, which can bring on feelings of immaturity and insecurity for being behind where I, or society, thinks I should be in life. Then, I was diagnosed with cancer. I felt as though God was saying, "Now, you focus on *this*!" My focus was completely redirected, and I realized that most of those fears were irrational, and I needed to concentrate on the "here and now" of my life.

I do not fear death. I did not fear my cancer as a death sentence. My faith in God is the reason for that. But, being a Christian does not guarantee a life without hardships or fear. There were many times the treatment journey was unbelievably scary! I talk about some of those in the following pages. My friend Stephanie sent bouquets of pink flowers at the beginning and end of radiation. She asked me on the last day if I had ever had any fear during the journey. Immediately, I responded, "Of course! But, it was that fear that made me more honest to God, others and myself about how I felt."

Most of the fear of my cancer stemmed from not knowing how treatment was going to go or how it would make me feel. God already knows how we feel, but He still wants us to talk to Him and be honest. Talking about it helped me lessen the fear and process what I was going through. I still need to talk about it sometimes.

Lord, thank You for giving me the strength to talk to others about my journey. I pray that may lessen their fears. Amen.

~~~

Day 4

"A merry heart doeth good like a medicine."
Proverbs 17:22 KJV

Before my readers get ready to throw this book at me, I need to put in a disclaimer. There is absolutely *nothing* funny about cancer. However, humor can help in the toughest situations. Prior to cancer, I was a positive but serious person most of the time. When I began this journey, everything changed. I became more positive...but less serious. Suddenly, I found things funny that I never thought would be! It was like hearing a really bad comedian and laughing one's head off just to get rid of a bunch of stress. I did that a lot!

I tried to stay positive and make others laugh. I realize now that I was not nearly as funny as I thought! I said a lot of things that I never thought I would say. I will share a list of some of those in more detail with you on the following pages. Hopefully, you will find some of them funny. You may find some of them appalling! Here is the list:

1. "I have breast cancer."
2. "I want my shirt to say, 'My titties are pretty!'"
3. "Yeah, I had another boob check today."
4. "That's interesting. I have a needle sticking out of my boob!"

5. "I'm getting my cup chipped!" (what I said to Mom right before my breast conservation surgery)
6. "Ooh, pretty!" (upon seeing my incision after surgery)
7. "I'm not dying! I've got breast cancer!"
8. "What do I care what he sees? He's done surgery on my boob!"
9. "Yeah, I remember him. He stuck a needle in my boob once."

Lord, thank You for giving us reasons to laugh! Thank You for having a sense of humor. Amen.

~~~

Day 5

"I want my shirt to say, 'My titties are pretty!'"

This whirlwind journey began within two hours of receiving my diagnosis. I had talked to each of my parents at least once, an oncologist was recommended, appointments were scheduled with the oncologist and a surgeon to discuss options, and my best friend Meg called me because she had already heard what she referred to as, "the annoying news." I had no time to react! Mom taught me that at times like these it is best to be proactive at first, and that there will be time to cry and be angry later. So, it was time to immediately act on the information I was receiving.

The appointment with my oncologist was the next day, so Mom made a quick trip to my home to go with me. I think it was helpful that both of us, while shocked, did our best to be proactive and not reactive. We discussed later that the oncologist had probably not seen many people appear so calm during an initial appointment.

Have you seen those shirts with pink ribbons on them that people wear for breast cancer awareness, or maybe because they have survived breast cancer and are literally wearing their excitement on their sleeve? I call them "survivor" shirts. Well, while we were eating lunch after my appointment I exclaimed to Mom in my 'I am going to survive this!' mood, "I want my [survivor] shirt to say, 'My titties are pretty!'" Let me give you a piece of advice. Never say that to your mother in the middle of a not-so-crowded Arby's restaurant where she can hear you! This was one of our favorite places. However, I think she was a bit embarrassed that I was with her at that moment. She said she was sure there are shirts that say nicer things than *that*! I'll let you be the judge as to whether mine was nicer. More on that later.

Lord, I pray that people reading this right now are laughing! Amen.

~~~

<u>Day 6</u>

"I have breast cancer!"

It was impressed upon me at an early age that there is a proper way to deliver bad news. If you wait until you have accepted the news yourself, say it clearly and with full voice, people are more likely to receive the news better than if you are upset when you tell them...or so I've been told. I also learned at a young age that sometimes there is no easy way to deliver bad news. Being diagnosed with cancer was one of those times. I was by myself when I received the news over the phone. I didn't have an immediate emotional reaction. My first thought was, "There are so many things that don't matter as much anymore!" But, that's beside the point.

In preparation for sharing the news with others, I took a minute to sit alone. I repeated the phrase...

I have breast cancer.
I have breast cancer.
I have breast cancer.

Once I could finally exclaim, "*Wow! I have breast cancer!*" out of a place of fact, not fear or nervous excitement, I felt as though I was ready to share the news with others. My neighbor Doug was a good friend who worked from home so was often there if I needed something…but it was his nap time, so I refrained from waking him up. I don't know why…but I never told him.

Several people knew I was going to have a biopsy, so I knew they would be as anxiously awaiting the results as I had been. Mom was with me for the procedure but had to go home to go back to her job before we knew what the biopsy revealed. My parents were divorced and living in separate states, so I had to tell each of them separately in the same way that I found out - over the phone.

Usually, I want to tell people *everything*, so I was not shy about it. I knew that telling other people that their daughter had breast cancer would help Mom and Dad process it, so I allowed them to tell several people on their own. Mom told Shane. She said he questioned whether the result was a false positive. I was glad to have Mom and Dad share the news with others because they could talk about it with other family members and friends in a way we could not at the time.

The announcement was easier sometimes than at other times. Telling my story is still that way. I never wanted anyone to pity me when I told them the news, so I would often follow up the announcement by holding my hand up as if I was telling them to wait before they reacted. Then I would say, "But, I'm fine!" I even made the announcement once or twice by saying, "I'm surviving breast cancer!" I have learned that how I say something may make absolutely *no* difference in how the news is received and I am learning to accept that.

One of the first people I told, after telling Mom and Dad, was Grandpa Roy. He is one of the first ones I want to inform about important life events, so I was glad Mom and I had already made plans to go see him and take him to a family gathering the following weekend.

Face-to-face conversations with Grandpa are often easier than phone conversations, so I waited until we arrived. I waited until Mom went out to the van to bring our luggage in so I could tell him while we were alone. I had to encourage Mom to go ahead and go outside...but she finally did. Grandpa can deal with most news calmly and make everyone else feel at ease. I have often called him my "It's gonna be alright" man, because he has exclaimed that sentiment, or a variation thereof, to me many times...calming my fear.

Grandpa Roy and I have often had difficult discussions while playing Cribbage because it seems easy to talk over the board. This time we were just sitting, talking. We were able to remain calm. We held hands as I told him, and he calmly told me he was "sorry to hear that." We talked some more before company that he was expecting that evening arrived.

Thinking back with my mind's ear, I can remember some of the rest of the conversation. Other parts of it are not as clear as they once were. I think he asked me about treatment for my cancer. I knew I might have to have chemo and radiation, but I had just received the news two days prior, so I explained to him that I was going to have more testing to get an exact diagnosis and see what proper treatment would be. I believe he also said, "Well, I hope everything works out for you with that...and I think it will! I'll be thinking of you and keeping you in my prayers." See what I mean about his attitude?

His overnight guests arrived. They had been longtime friends of my grandparents and were a delightful couple! The visit was a much-needed distraction. They took us out to dinner, and we had a nice time getting to know one another. We got back home to Grandpa's house and I said goodnight and hugged Grandpa and my new friends and went to bed. In the morning one of my new friends, Mary, said to me, "I don't know exactly what is going on, but I know you are going through something, and I want to give you this." She had traveled with a little box of blank cards with beautiful pink flowers on them but had no plans of doing anything with them.

The cards were perfect for many "Thank-You's" I needed to write. Of course, I sent one to her, explaining what was going on. I'm glad I told her. I kept the box after using the cards so I could keep other nice notes and keepsakes in it that I received during treatment.

Lord, please help the people reading this right now who have bad news to share, share their news in whatever way works for them. Amen.

~~~

<u>Day 7</u>

What cancer CANNOT do

I met my radiation oncologist early in the journey so I could make a well-informed decision as to a plan of action. The appointment was right after lunchtime and I arrived before the receptionists' office had opened back up. Finally, I had some time to react to the news. I looked around the room and there on the wall was a framed copy of part of a poem called *Cancer is So Limited*. It inspired me greatly! I had never seen the poem before, but soon it became my favorite.

A couple of years after treatment I looked up the poem and found it in a book self-published by the author. I was showing it to Dad and the lady he was dating at the time. She happened to be in a poetry guild and when she saw the author's name she said, "I know him!" She sent his contact information to me. Though I thought it was a long shot, I wrote him a letter asking for permission to use the poem. He wrote back and graciously gave me permission to use his poem in my book.

Cancer Is So Limited

They've sentenced you with invisible cells that secrete
themselves deep in body recesses and multiply
lymphatic assault on vital functions.

Can cancer conquer you?
I doubt it, for the strengths I see in you have
nothing to do with cells and blood and muscle.

For cancer is so limited...
It cannot cripple love.
It cannot shatter hope.
It cannot corrode faith.
It cannot eat away peace.
It cannot destroy confidence.
It cannot kill friendship.
It cannot shut out memories.
It cannot silence courage.
It cannot invade the soul.
It cannot steal eternal life.
It cannot quench the spirit.
It cannot cancel resurrection.

Can cancer conquer you?
I doubt it, for the strengths I see in you have
nothing to do with cells and blood and muscle.

Robert L. Lynn[1]

---

[1] Lynn, R. L. (2013) Cancer is so Limited and Other Poems of Faith. United States. CreateSpace

Lord, thank You that cancer is so limited. Amen.

~ ~ ~

<u>Day 8</u>

Decisions...decisions

After finding out more about the exact diagnosis I was able to make informed decisions about the next steps to take. I don't need to bore you with the details, but they made a difference as to which cancer surgery I was going to have done.

When I was first learning about the diagnosis I decided that if a mastectomy was a good option, I would go with it. I didn't care how that would make me look. When I gathered information from all the doctors involved in my care, I was informed that a mastectomy was not necessary. I was kind of relieved. The surgery is more serious than some would think. With the medical issues I was already experiencing, there were more risks of doing an unnecessary surgery, (i.e., longer recuperation time).

I know many women who had mastectomies or double mastectomies for various reasons. That was the right decision for them. Some are urged to make that decision. I commend them as well. An important thing to remember if you are on this journey too, is, despite all the guidance you may receive regarding the decision, it is *your* decision and only *yours*. It is your body and you have to live with whatever happens to it. Don't let anyone ever tell you any different! It is one of the hardest and most important decisions of your life and it, along with the diagnosis, will change it forever. Make sure you know enough to make an informed decision...and make it.

Considering all the information I had gathered, I made the informed decision that breast-conserving surgery, A.K.A., a lumpectomy to remove the lump, was the best option for me. The surgeon agreed.

Lord, please help the ones reading this who are trying to make this important decision. Amen.

~~~

Day 9

"Yeah, I had another boob check today".

Some of us were not born with much modesty. Sometimes modesty becomes less important as one gets older. My extensive medical history has not allowed me to have much modesty. In fact, I feel as though I am not allowed much at all in the doctor's office. What little modesty I had left flew out the window when I was diagnosed with cancer.

Whatever may be the case for you, once one has been diagnosed with breast cancer one often gets used to talking about breasts. Some may call them breasts, tits, titties, etc. I got used to talking about my boobs. I had a lot of "boob checks" (breast exams) - most of them done by male doctors and nurses with whom I became very comfortable. Again, that is a personal choice you need to make.

Being inexperienced with self-breast exams prior to finding the lump, I had to learn a lot about how my boobs were supposed to feel. I used to find it kind of uncomfortable to talk about breasts. Women need to learn to get over this discomfort. We need to know how our bodies are supposed to feel. Our male counterparts need to learn how their bodies are supposed to feel as well. Although it is not as common, men can also get breast cancer. Men and women can get various forms of cancer, and if we don't know how our bodies are supposed to feel, we will not be able to detect when there is a problem.

I like to use the phrase "have the conversation." Having the conversation about certain checks for cancer may help save a life someday. That life may be yours. That life may be that of a dear friend or family member. At the chagrin of some of my friends and family, I have become one of those women who enjoys having a nice relaxing conversation about cancer in the middle of a crowded coffee shop or restaurant. If you do not yet have one of these women in your life...find her. If you want to know how to become one of those women…find me. Shoot! Find me anyway. I would love to talk with you!

Lord, thank you for giving me comfort in telling my story so that I may help others have the conversation. Amen.

~ ~ ~

<u>Day 10</u>

The plan of action

My treatment plan originally included four sessions of chemotherapy each three weeks apart, a six-week break, and thirty-three days of radiation. After healing from the lumpectomy, I had a port-a-cath inserted to make chemo easier. A port-a-cath, or port, is "a device used to draw blood and give treatments, including intravenous fluids, drugs, or blood transfusions. The port is placed under the skin, usually in the chest. It is attached to a catheter (a thin, flexible tube) that is guided (threaded) into a large vein above the right side of the heart called the superior vena cava. A port-a-cath may stay in place for many weeks or months" (NCI Dictionary of Cancer Terms, n.d.).

In order to use the port, a phlebotomist certified in "accessing" the port must be available.

"Accessing" simply means to put a needle into the port and inject a couple of solutions to open the catheter. After that is done the port is supposed to produce what is called "blood return", blood coming from the vein and returning out of the port. Usually this is an easy process for most people. I am not most people!

The first use of my port was to be for an iron infusion that the doctor said I needed to increase my iron before chemo. The port was accessed but it did not return blood. I was getting the injection in the hospital. Luckily, my surgeon happened to be there. He checked it and was able to flush saline into and out of it just fine. But, the nurses had to follow protocol, so I was sent immediately to the radiology department to make sure the port had not moved.

The radiologist said it was still in place but would not and may never return blood...so...I had the infusion intravenously (in other words, through a needle that was poked into a vein and hooked up to a long plastic tube), and it went well. Although the port didn't return blood at the hospital that day, it did return blood for chemo and bloodwork *after* treatment. As for bloodwork *during* treatment, that's another story for another day.

Lord, thank You for things that are supposed to make our lives easier, even if they seem to make our lives harder at times. Amen.

~~~

<u>Day 11</u>

"There is no sound advice." - Krista Wilke Ranby

I wrote to Krista during my journey with cancer to let her know what an inspiration she is. She's an amazing woman! Krista was in graduate school pursuing a Ph.D. in Social Psychology when she was diagnosed with cancer, obtained the degree, and started a family within a few years of her diagnosis and treatment!

I wish I had had that much ambition during treatment! Most of the time I felt good about conjuring up enough energy to do laundry, but that was about it. I did a lot of laundry, but that's beside the point. When Krista wrote back to me, she gave me the quote mentioned above.

Everyone has an opinion about cancer. When I found out that I had it, I found out that everyone also had advice on how I should handle it. Most of them had *no business* giving that advice. Some did, but told me based on their experience, not mine. Now I get to talk about it through my experience, but I know it happens differently for everyone.

I heard it all, but I learned to discern what I was hearing. A nurse practitioner, who was a former oncology nurse, told me everything she knew about cancer...before knowing all the facts about *my* cancer. She was guessing why my cancer occurred and told me what *could* happen. I know she meant well, but she told me all this right before my first appointment with the oncologist, and it scared the daylights out of me! To top it all off, at least half of what she told me ended up not applying to my type of cancer. Mom was with me for that appointment and I could tell that she too was overwhelmed by information overload!

I learned that peoples' advice was often coming from their opinions about cancer, not always the truth. God taught me to listen to my body first, oncology doctors and nurses second, and others who have or have had cancer third. Even dentists and eye doctors will discuss possible side effects of chemo. Hearing about these effects is scary, but I listened because I wanted to be aware of what they might feel like and how to combat them. This worked well for me.

I also learned that just because side effects are *possible* does not mean they are *probable*. I will readily talk about what worked for me, especially when someone is seeking a suggestion, but I know that every diagnosis is as individual as the person who received it. If you must go through it, you do what works for you.

There was a series of conversations that I loved because they were not advice at all...they were encouragement and understanding from Rachael who is another one of my best friends. She and I have been friends since kindergarten. She sent cards to me at least once every other week during treatment. I don't know where she found them, but they were the best gifts I could have received! They talked about cancer and the journey. They talked about how much cancer *sucks*. They told me that cancer is tough...but I'm tougher!

Sometimes Rachael would send a "Thinking of you" card or pictures that her daughters colored for me, but the "cancer" cards were my favorites because that let me know it was okay to talk to her about what I was going through. We texted back and forth and messaged on Facebook or e-mailed periodically, but those cards were conversations in and of themselves, and I appreciated them immensely!

Lord, I pray that if my readers are going through cancer treatment, they may have as easy a time as I did. Most of all, I pray that You teach them to learn to discern and I thank You for helping me do so. I'm sorry for the times I do not want to listen. Amen.

~~~

<u>Day 12</u>

*"Birthdays are good for you. Statistics show that
the people who have the most live the longest."
- Father Larry Lorenzoni*

I celebrated my thirty-sixth birthday two
weeks before my first chemo treatment. Boy, what a
celebration! I decided I loved pink, so I had a pink
cake and pink decorations. I was getting so used to
telling people I had breast cancer that I was loving the
conversations - and tended to go overboard with
them. For example, I wanted a pink ribbon on my
cake. Mom suggested that I shouldn't have that
because I should want people to be happy to see me
because they wanted to celebrate with me, not just
because I had breast cancer. I agreed.

I was able to have this wonderful party at my
church the day before my birthday and had a few
conversations about breast cancer. A good friend of
mine gave several little gifts to me with the pink
breast cancer ribbon on them. They were special too
because I wanted to be able to acknowledge that I had
it without other people feeling as though it was taboo
to talk about.

Saying I had cancer is not as important as, I
like to say, "having the conversation." Sometimes
the conversation was about mammograms.
Sometimes it was about cancer, and I had the
opportunity to find out that some of my longtime

friends from the church were survivors. Some of those wonderful conversations were not about cancer. I was able to see friends that I had not seen in a long time, meet their children, and be surrounded by incredibly special people whom I love.

I had so much fun! Birthdays are special anyway, but every birthday I celebrate as a cancer survivor is an extra special one. I just wish it did not take cancer to help me realize that celebrating birthdays is so special.

Lord, thank you for giving us days to celebrate. Amen.

~~~

Day 13

Because He Lives

Hearing about possible side effects of chemo and radiation was nerve-racking! When I tried to remember that just because the side effects *could* happen didn't mean they *would*, I was more at peace about treatment. There was no doubt I was going to go through with it, so worrying about it did not do any good.

Shortly before my treatments started, I decided I was excited to find out what chemo would do to my body. My treatments were on Mondays, so

I attended church regularly the day before. I will never forget being in church the day before my first treatment. The organist played two of my favorite hymns. This one also happened to be Mom's favorite hymn. I find the chorus to be especially meaningful.

"Because He Lives"

"God sent His son, they called Him Jesus
He came to love, heal and forgive
He lived and died to buy my pardon
An empty grave is there to prove my Savior lives

Because He lives, I can face tomorrow
Because He lives, all fear is gone
Because I know He holds the future
and life is worth the living, just because He lives

How sweet to hold a newborn baby
and feel the pride and joy He gives
But greater still the calm assurance
this child can face uncertain day because He lives

Because He lives, I can face tomorrow
Because He lives, all fear is gone
Because I know He holds the future
and life is worth the living, just because He lives

And then one day, I'll cross the river
I'll fight life's final war with pain
and then, as death gives way to victory

I'll see the lights of glory and I'll know He reigns

Because He lives, I can face tomorrow
Because He lives, all fear is gone
Because I know He holds the future
and life is worth the living, just because He lives

Because He lives, I can face tomorrow
Because He lives, all fear is gone
Because I know He holds the future
and life is worth the living, just because He lives

Because He lives, I can face tomorrow.
Because He lives all fear is gone.
Because I know He holds the future
and life is worth the living, just because He lives."

Bill and Gloria Gaither[2]

Lord, thank You that we can face tomorrow because You live. Please help the ladies and gentlemen who are reading this know that You live. Amen.

~ ~ ~

[2] Gaither, G. and Gaither, W. (1971) Because He Lives

<u>Day 14</u>

"I'm not dying! I've got breast cancer!"

As much as I have loved some of the conversations regarding cancer, there were those I hated. One was with a friend who was one of my personal care attendants, so I saw her daily and we talked a lot. She had had indirect experience with cancer. In other words, she had not had cancer herself but had several family members and friends who had cancer. Some of them passed away.

She shared with me that she believed all of us have cancer inside our bodies and that somehow, we do something that "turns it on" and makes us sick. She also thought chemo made everyone receiving it extremely sick. I took the first statement as accusatory, and the second one seemed too much of a generalization. Right or wrong, her views came from her experience.

I decided early in the journey to announce my diagnosis by stating that I was surviving breast cancer. I answered the general question of, "How are you?" with "I'm surviving!" That is, until the day of this conversation.

As I was trying to be positive about the cancer, my friend said, "And I do hope you survive this." Thinking of it now, this was a nice, caring statement. However, I did not take it that way at the time. I received her statement as if she did not have the faith that I did that I was going to survive. I said to myself, "That's not what I said!" I snapped at my friend - yes, you guessed it - "I'm not dying! I've got breast cancer!"

Now, before you decide to beat me with this book, I know that breast cancer can be fatal, even after the first battle. I've lost friends to breast cancer. I know how sick treatment can make some people. I also know how treatable it can be in some cases. Personally, I never looked at my diagnosis as a death sentence and had faith that God was going to let me survive *this* time.

Grandma Dorothy passed away after having ovarian cancer several years prior to my diagnosis. Shortly before I started my own treatment for cancer, my Grandma Marjorie passed away after having Alzheimer's Disease. I love and miss each of them more than words can say, and I know I will see both again in Heaven someday. But, immediately after receiving my diagnosis I remember thinking of Grandma Marjorie and saying under my breath, "Sorry Grandma, I'm not joining you anytime soon!"

I declared that I was surviving breast cancer whenever I could. The care package that Aunt Roma sent also included several craft projects. I guess she knew I was about to have a lot of time on my hands! Anyway, there were a few wooden pieces that I could paint, some cool Sharpie paint pens and some magnets to put on the back of the wooden pieces.

I don't remember what I painted for Dad...but I painted two pieces. For Mom, I painted a butterfly and a flower. I painted an "M" for myself. All, of course, in pink. On the back of each of the wooden pieces, I wrote a big bold statement. For Mom and Dad, "My daughter is surviving breast cancer!" For me, "I am surviving breast cancer!" I had also written that the hot pink journal belonged to: "A breast cancer survivor!" I expected everyone else to believe that I was going to survive, and I was bound and determined to drill it into their heads.

    To my relief, after I was diagnosed, my friend never mentioned her belief that everyone already has cancer inside again. She did mention the day before my first chemo treatment that "chemo is going to make you sick, sick, sick!" I reminded her quickly that we didn't know that for sure. Maybe seeing me go through it changed her views. Maybe not. All I know is that we did not talk about my cancer much after that conversation. Not being able to talk to her about such a huge part of my life was hard since I saw her daily.

    In addition, I decided to quit telling people, "I'm surviving." I wish I had never let that discussion change me in that way.

Lord, please help us stay truthful in our conversations. Help us to be more influenced by You instead of the world in what we do and say. Amen.

~~~

<u>Day 15</u>

"I don't like your attitude!"

Several months before I was diagnosed with cancer, I began experiencing what counselors call "compassion fatigue." I was practicing as a counselor at the time, but unfortunately, I was burnt out, and did not have the heart to hear about some of my clients' issues. I would listen but think, "You have no idea what I'm going through!" I was not at that job very long.

One of the ladies in my cancer support group at First United Methodist Church in Manhattan Kansas, advised me that since I had been diagnosed, I had permission to say to people, "I don't like your attitude!" I hate to admit it, but I was a little too good at that...even with family.

I have tried to maintain a positive attitude all my life in order to help other people not feel sorry for me. I reached a point, even before the diagnosis, in which I expected everyone around me to keep a positive attitude. After all, it can be said that positive people attract positive people, right? So, this worked...sometimes.

If there is anything *negative* about always being *positive* it is that I stopped wanting to listen to people talk about their problems. I hated myself for feeling that way! I have grown up loving to listen to people tell me all their problems! Wait...that came out wrong. I don't love the fact that others have problems. I love having people talk to me! I love gaining trust from somebody that will sit down and tell me their life stories...problems and all.

I was at a point in my life in which everyone else's problems seemed to pale in comparison to the ones I was having. If someone had a major issue, I understood. If the issue didn't seem major it was as though people were crying because they had hangnails! I felt like saying to them, "Oh wa, quit complaining!" That was when I realized...I had hit rock bottom.

I know I am not always the cheeriest person to be around. Talking about medical issues of others (or my own) has always given me a way to process what was going on, and I do so with ease. This is not always conducive to being positive, and I tried to keep that in mind. If people tired of or were resistant to talking about my cancer, I stopped.

I must remind myself occasionally that others have gone through far worse than I. I have learned that my positivity does not always help someone else remain positive. I have also learned that others are entitled to their feelings and I should not try to change or dismiss them.

I am the one who needs an attitude adjustment. I remember sitting in my apartment one day after a grueling day of treatment.

Suddenly, I heard a voice ask, "Do you get it now"?!
Yes, Lord, I get it.

Lord, thank You for helping me change my attitude.
Help those of us who expect others to keep us happy.
Amen.

~~~

Day 16

Time to see what happens

September 15, 2014 was my first day of chemo. I was blessed to have Mom with me so she could help me listen to the nurses and be aware of how I was feeling. I listened as all the known side effects were explained to me. I paid attention to what could be done to combat them so that I would know what to do if I experienced one or more of them. My port was easily accessed and decided to return blood this time!

The medication was given by an IV pump and the rate that the first medication dripped could be set manually or automatically. This proved to be important to remember because the first time I was given this, the rate was automatically set to 150, almost the fastest rate that could be set for the average adult, which I am *not*. I was blessed to be aware that this was too fast for my body. My heart rate rose quickly, and I started to feel light-headed and just downright wonky. One of the chemo nurses was immediately by my side. In no time at all, all four nurses in the treatment room tended to me and were ready to give me oxygen. I was sitting up, fully alert and speaking, but the oxygen meter was not able to read my oxygen level. That was terrifying for the nurses and confusing for me!

The doctor was called immediately, and medication was stopped. I was given two anti-nausea medications through the port. The rate was reset manually and started again at the slowest rate possible. This increased the duration of each treatment from two to four hours, but I didn't care. It worked at the slower rate, and I did not feel as though I was going to pass out! Low and slow was just fine with me.

I had moved to Junction City after my diagnosis to be closer to family. While I was living in Junction City, Grandpa called often to see if he could bring me lunch and come play games for a while. He called that day just as Mom and I were getting back to my place. As tired as I was, I can never say *no* to Grandpa, so he came over and the three of us had a good lunch and games that afternoon. He also brought some beautiful roses to me. Mom took a picture of me holding the roses and said I looked so good I *did not* look like I had just had chemo. I always try to look better than I feel. Mission accomplished!

Grandpa's energy level is also amazing! He really helped me through this exhausting time in my life by visiting me at least once a week and taking me to Sunday school and church almost every Sunday. Having his company meant so much to me!

Lord, thank You for making me aware of my body and giving me the strength to talk about how I am feeling. I pray You give that strength to the ladies and gentlemen reading this. Amen.

~~~

Day 17

Have the conversation

Ever since I was diagnosed, I have had some of the most wonderful conversations with people who had cancer. One such conversation occurred before my second chemo treatment. Dad and I were in the waiting room, and a gentleman came in with his family. We said hello to each other as he came in and went back to the treatment room.

I was still in the waiting room when he returned. I noticed him opening the door for his family so they could leave, but he did not follow them. Instead, he approached me by standing in front of me. I said hello to him again. Somehow, he knew that I, not my dad, was the cancer patient, and he preceded to ask about my cancer.

Many cancer patients learn to be open with each other, so I answered him freely. Likewise, he described his cancer in detail, such as where it was, his treatment plan, and so on. His next statement was something to the effect of, "I think God gives us cancer so that we can learn to love each other and others in a way that we might not otherwise."

Wow! What a witness! I agree with him on so many levels. I wouldn't say that I have more sympathy for those with cancer, but I have more empathy towards them. After having gone through it myself I know so much more about cancer and its effects.

I will never pretend to know *exactly* what someone else with cancer is going through, but I know what I went through and how I felt while going through it. I do not think that a person must go through everything personally to be empathetic towards someone going through something difficult. However, I now see that in some cases, it helps.

I have no idea who or where this man is today, but I pray that he is doing well, and I know he is praising God wherever he may be. He said something I could never put into words and really made me think. I am not sure God *gives* us diseases. I do believe that He gives us trials so He can help us through them and make us better on the other side of the trial.

Lord, thank You for that gentleman and his family. Amen.

~ ~ ~

<u>Day 18</u>

"If at first you don't succeed...try...try again!"
- Thomas H. Palmer

Precautions were taken so I would not have the same reaction to chemo the second time as I did the first time. I was blessed to have Dad with me this time. Dad always finds a way to bring humor, positivity and calmness into a difficult situation. I was a rather serious child with an old soul, so I did not always appreciate that he could find humor in a lot of things, but the older I get, the more I appreciate that he still can.

I wouldn't have had any problems for the second treatment, *except,* the nurse who set the rate for the first medication accidentally set it automatically instead of manually. So, it was started at the same speed as before. Once again, my body negatively reacted quickly. All I could do was raise my hand, and after seeing me do that, Dad asked me if it was happening again. I nodded, and he immediately alerted the nurses. Now...keep in mind...he was not with me for my first reaction, he had only heard about it. Way to go Dad! After that nurse realized what she had done, she claimed she didn't know *how* that happened! But, that's beside the point.

The medication was stopped, the rate slowed, and I was fine after it was restarted at the correct rate. Dad realized that we could see the rate on the machine ourselves so from that day on I turned the machine towards me so I could watch it. The nurse that made the mistake during my second chemo treatment was not allowed to touch me until it was time for the medications that were given at a "flat," or preset rate. After her mistake, she was just as nice as she could be every time I saw her!

After treatment was over for the day, Dad took me to one of our favorite places for lunch, Olive Garden. He has taught me to always learn and remember the waitstaffs' name, and most of the time he introduces us to them as well.

I still remember the waitress we had that day. Her name is Hensley. She came to our table with the complimentary bottle of wine they always try to get people to sample and asked if there was anything special that we were celebrating that day. I told her I guessed we were celebrating that I just finished my second chemo treatment. At the time, I thought that was halfway through, so I probably told her that too. She congratulated me. At the end of the meal she did something that meant so much to me. As the waitstaff often does, she gave Dad a card with her name and a thank you for dining there. He read it and said, "Here, I think this is for you." She wrote a nice note wishing me well with chemo and a great week. I got a chance to thank her and kept the note in my special box.

Lord, thank You for helping me through this. I pray that those going through chemo right now have as easy a time with it as possible. I pray that they can handle whatever happens. Amen.

~~~

Day 19

Hair today...gone tomorrow

I began to lose my hair before the second chemo treatment. I don't consider myself a vain person. It's even hard for me to remember to comb my hair if I am going to see someone, because I usually don't care much about my physical image. So, when I thought about losing my hair, I did not think I would care about how that would look.

I mentioned in a cancer support group meeting that I was not considering covering my head as I lost my hair. One of the ladies said, "Sweetheart, your head's going to get cold!" I hadn't thought about that. I was losing my hair during a chilly fall and winter. In October of that year, a wig was donated to the group, and it was decided that I should have it since everyone else had passed that point in their treatments. The concerned lady that warned me about the cold, donated leftover shampoo and conditioner she had used for her wig. I can remember Grandpa Ralph jokingly saying that he enjoyed when Grandma Dorothy started to wear a wig because all he had to do was take *her wig* to the beauty parlor to get fixed. He didn't have to take *her*. He was so funny! Grandma Dorothy's hair grew back in as beautiful, thick and curly as ever just before she passed away. That gave me hope when I had to wear a wig...which incidentally never got to go to the beauty parlor!

As soon as I decided to accept the wig and other head coverings, my hair started to fall out...*rapidly!* Who'd a thunk it? I received the wig and found out it was blonde. Someone told me it was brown with blonde highlights. Trust me...it was *blonde*!

After trying it on for the first time I took a few silly selfies and sent one to Mom. I called immediately after sending the picture to see what she thought. She answered the phone, "Hello, Marilyn!" (referring to Marilyn Monroe). I showed the wig to Grandpa Roy before putting any pictures on social media. As soon as I put a picture on social media, Aunt Bonnie, Mom's youngest sister, commented, "Well, *hello*, Marilyn!" Mom and her sisters often thought alike, but that was pretty funny!

The wig wasn't quite *that* blonde, but I did dress up as Goldilocks and the three bears for Halloween. If I would have still had the wig by Halloween the following year, I was going to dress as the iconic actress, but I did not so I could not.

I have been a brunette since birth and had decided to always be happy with the hair color God gave me. However, when I began losing my hair I decided that, if God was going to let that happen, perhaps He would be okay if I played with the color a bit. So, as I like to say, chemo made me a beautiful blonde! As I wore the wig proudly that fall and winter I sang, "I've got a new added do!" (instead of "new attitude"), and "I've got my wig to keep me warm!" (instead of "I've got my love to keep me warm!")

I was never good at putting on head scarves. I had several hats I liked to wear with or without the wig. I hated hats, but I had a few that were pink or another pretty color or pattern that I would wear if I needed my head covered for warmth. I remember the first time I wore a hat to church. It was one that I really liked that was leopard print. I had not yet worn my wig out in public, so I decided to try this hat first to see how people would react.

All I had to do was mention chemo to my pastor at church, and he would stop, pardon the pun "at the drop of a hat," and sit down next to me in the pew to talk. As the pastor walked by me in church that Sunday and asked how I was doing I said, "baldness is *much* sexier on a man!" That got his attention! He stopped, sat down, agreed with me, and said, "You sure are sportin' that hat!" I really appreciated him and his willingness to talk.

My friend Sheila, whom I will mention again later, disagreed with me that baldness is much sexier on a man. I don't know if she was just trying to make me feel better, but I wasn't sure she knew what she was talking about because her husband appeared to have a full head of hair! Hmmm, I wonder what he looks like now? I learned to enjoy my new style and care a little more about what I looked like.

Lord, thank You that chemo made me a beautiful blonde for a while. Amen.

~~~

Day 20

I thought I was done

As I mentioned earlier, my chemo ended up going a little *too* well, if that's possible. I had to have bloodwork done every week. My blood counts were usually normal, partially due to the medications I was on before and after treatment. My usually atypical body was handling treatment much better than many people, including myself, thought it would. The original plan was to have four chemo treatments, take a six-week break to let my body adjust, then have radiation. Treatments were once a week, every three weeks, and I had appointments with the oncologist on the weeks I did not have treatment.

When I saw the doctor prior to the fourth treatment, we discussed the fact that my body was responding so well. I was so excited because I thought I was almost done! Just as I expressed this to the doctor, he asked me, "How about two more chemo treatments?" My excitement quickly subsided. The doctor explained that he had ordered four chemo at a very low dosage to see how I would tolerate them, but that studies showed that at least six chemo treatments for my type of cancer are better than just four. There was a weekend between the appointment and the fourth treatment, so he asked me to think about it over the weekend and agreed to do the same.

I remember telling Mom about the conversation. She said that didn't seem like much of a reward for treatment going well! I agreed, but we knew I had to pray and think about it. I did a lot of both that weekend. I cannot explain it in this book, but I always knew when Mom was praying for me and could tell that she also did a lot of praying that weekend also.

I thought about Brandon who had always had a tough time with chemo but took it anyway to treat his cancer. I decided that if he could do it, I could do it.

When I saw the doctor in the treatment room the following Monday, he walked over to me. Before he could say anything, I put my hand up and asked, "Okay, before you give me your decision, did you *pray* about it?" Immediately he said yes, and that was all I needed in order to accept his answer. He also mentioned talking to some of his friends (I assumed he meant colleagues in oncology) and they agreed with him that additional treatments were needed. I appreciated that he was willing to consult the Great Physician and his own colleagues. That is the mark of a good doctor. He recommended two more treatments and I agreed. The treatments went well, and I was confident that the correct decision was made.

Lord, thank You for being in that decision. Amen.

~~~

<u>Day 21</u>

Thirty-three days of pink!

The last two chemotherapy treatments happened without any "hiccups" as my oncologist put it, and I celebrated being done for real this time! Dad went with me to my last treatment, so I am sure we celebrated at Olive Garden again.

I was still given six weeks between chemo and radiation to take a break and find out what was going to happen to my body after that phase of treatment, during which time, I continued to be a beautiful blonde. Just when I thought my neuropathy (sudden tingling and numbness of hands and/or feet that is common with chemo) was gone I was occasionally reminded that it was still there. It was crazy to be able to hold my cell phone in my right hand and suddenly have it jump across me and fall on the floor to my left! Other than some occasional numbness, I felt great! I had energy that I hadn't felt in several months!

I decided to take time to purposefully reorganize my closet. It seemed to be the proper thing to do to wear pink to each appointment regarding my cancer. So, to prepare for radiation, I arranged my closet for "twenty-five days of pink!" Yes, I *did* own that much pink, and yes, it is *way* too much pink!

I saw my radiation oncologist weekly while going through radiation. When I had my first appointment with him after a few days of radiation he subtracted the number of days I had done with a certain number. Wait, did he subtract right? What he subtracted would make my days of radiation add up to thirty-three, not twenty-five. What?! He was quick to remind me that I was to have thirty-three days of radiation, not just twenty-five. Here we go again with more treatment than I expected. I'm sure I had that written down somewhere, but remembering such details became more difficult. There was so much to remember! Anyway, I digress.

I added to my closet a bit, so the "thirty-three days of pink!" would be possible. I think the only pink article of over- or under- clothing that I didn't own at the time was a pair of shoes. I am a problem solver, so I tied pink hair ties to the zipper pulls of a pair of black shoes that I wore all the time. I kidded with one of the radiation therapists that I did it so that it was easier for them to see my black shoes as they put them on their black floor, but he was not amused.

It is much more fun to refer to my "thirty-three days of pink!" rather than radiation. I think I had to wear red instead of pink once or twice. Mom reminded me that, "Red is just a strong pink!"

I had to go for an appointment prior to beginning radiation so the doctor and radiation therapists could mark exactly where the radiation needed to go. I was also fitted with a special pillow that would aid in positioning during each treatment. Mom took me to the appointment but was not allowed back into the treatment room. She did not join me for any radiation treatments either but wore a pink ribbon every day for the duration. She told me to just think of it as getting glamour shots taken every day. The problem was, in that odd position, I felt about as glamourous as a fish!

Kate started to do the "thirty-three days of pink!" with me and encouraged others to do so. She would send me pictures of her pink on Facebook. Unfortunately, Kate became ill during this time and was not able to finish my pink days with me. She expressed to me that there were times during her illness she could not even get up to get dressed in the morning and that she felt more green than pink during some of those days. I dismissed her from showing me her pink (or green) for the rest of that time. Fortunately, she got through her illness and the last time I saw her she was doing great!

Lord, thank You for pink! Amen.

~~~

Day 22

God has a sense of humor!

I began "thirty-three days of pink" in February of 2015. I was still exhausted from all the chemo treatments and somewhat nervous about what radiation would do to my body. Something comical happened on the way to treatment for the first few days. I would hear a song on the radio and the next person or people that I saw would be dancing to that song. Funny thing was...they weren't really dancing!

I hear a lot of you saying, "Melody, you were seeing things!" or "Your mind was playing tricks on you!" I know it must seem like that. I tend to get annoyingly giggly when I am nervous, and I was probably so tired that I could have been seeing things that weren't happening. I say that it was God's humor. I tried to always enter treatment with a positive attitude although I dreaded radiation. The fact that I was seeing something amusing before I went in...that was God giving me humor to get through it.

Scott, one of the radiation therapists, was rather serious most of the time. In fact, I thought of him as stoic and was known to call him an 'ole stick in the mud' from time to time. So, I made it my mission every single day of radiation to try to make him laugh. I found out that his humor was a little cruder than mine was at the time. I remember one day when the three therapists were trying to set a measurement of some kind on the radiation machine. He was on one side of the machine and pushed a button that turned off something for one of the therapists on the other side. She said, "Hey! You turned me off!" With a smirk on his face he asked, "Are you saying I turn you on?!" The therapist he asked turned to me and said, "*That's* the kind of stuff that makes *him* laugh!" I did think what she said was kind of funny, although I was too much of a prude at the time to admit it.

My sense of humor changed when I was diagnosed. Some would even say I lost my filter. I guess I still had a little bit of a filter because I would never use crude humor just to make him laugh. I did make him giggle a few times and laugh once. Every day after getting me into position for radiation, the therapists would go back into a room that had three screens that they watched during radiation. I guess they showed where the radiation was hitting the affected areas. I noticed the screens one day and started calling them the "boob tube" since I was having radiation due to breast cancer.

I know, I *funny*...and a little *naughty*! I explained to Scott one day about the "boob tube" and he laughed out loud, stifling his laughter quickly as though he didn't want me to know I had actually succeeded in making him laugh. That was funny!

Trying to make Scott laugh was a fun game I played to make my life more fun during this time. I know that was God because I ended up getting along better with him than I did with the other therapists. I did not expect to feel more comfortable around male doctors and nurses for breast cancer treatment, but I was. Don't get me wrong. There are some excellent oncology nurses that are female, but I was uncomfortable being around some of them. Scott was nice and tried hard to make me as comfortable as possible.

"Thirty-three days of pink!" makes radiation sound more fun than it actually was. Truth is, it was grueling! I will explain why tomorrow. God uses humor to heal us sometimes and He got me through that phase of my treatment. It was typical of my radiation oncologist and I to laugh a lot during my weekly appointments. Again, that was God!

The easiest part about radiation was transportation to and from appointments. I lived in Junction City, Kansas at the time and my treatments were in Manhattan, Kansas. Luckily, my insurance pays for out-of-town trips to medical appointments if I let them set up the transportation. I became close friends with a woman named Tracy who owned one of the transportation services. At the time, her son Tristian helped her periodically and her son Marcus was another driver for the business. Tracy and/or one of her sons had picked me up for so many out-of-town appointments that we became close like family. They have even come to my rescue twice when my van was stranded somewhere and bought lunch for me on several occasions! Tristian and Marcus are much younger but much taller than I am (which really isn't saying much since I'm so short!), so I think of them as my big little brothers!

When it came time for me to start radiation, Tracy graciously offered to put it on her schedule so they could take me to all my radiation appointments...*all of them*! This was a load off my mind because I knew I could trust them. I never had to worry whether I would have the ride or be able to arrive safely on time, which made an otherwise frustrating aspect of treatment more manageable.

Marcus drove me to and from several of those appointments, especially for the last two weeks. There was a song that came on the radio one day while he was driving. I mentioned how much I *hated* that song. Of course, the song played on the radio almost every day after that...sometimes just as we were turning the corner to go to my place! Marcus would laugh so hard every time it came on! He even sang it to me one day and started calling it "our song" from that point forward. The song still makes me laugh! I can only hope he has a good time explaining that to his wife after she reads this. Gotcha Marcus!

God, thank You for humor and reminding us to laugh, even in difficult phases of our lives. Amen.

~~~

Day 23

Lessons in Melody's anatomy

I needed all that humor in order to get through radiation. I *hated* it! There, I said it. I *hated* it! It was not painful at all, but I did have some sore muscles after each treatment from having to stretch into that strange position and hold it for a few minutes. I had minimal side effects from the radiation itself.

The grueling part of it was that my body does not move like the average person's body. I have no voluntary movement in my lower extremities, so what should have been as simple as lying on the table and getting a little laser treatment was not simple at all. I found it rather odd that the technicians helping me and controlling the radiation were called "therapists". That was *not* what I would call therapeutic! Learning to work with three radiation therapists to move my body into an unnatural position safely was a constant struggle.

My legs are extremely fragile, so I have a habit of watching anytime they are handled by someone else. In order to get into the right position for radiation I had to lay flat on my back and let three strangers move my hips and legs *without* being able to watch what they were doing or have someone with me to watch and direct them. Honestly, it was terrifying in the beginning! This was unnatural for me and took a lot of trust that I didn't always have. It takes at least twenty days, some even say thirty, to form a habit. I had thirty-three days of radiation. *You* do the math!

Even the radiation therapist I got along with best argued that it was easier for them to get me into position than it was for me to do it myself. I took that as a challenge. I love challenges, but this one was not as fun as most of the challenges I have chosen to take on in life.

At the same time as I took on this challenge, I was dealing with some negativity from a few people I saw outside of treatment. I'm sure that didn't help my attitude any either. Other people believe I am so naturally kind and patient. *Trust me,* sometimes it is just an act!

Eventually, the therapists learned that I could get myself into position quicker than they could, and I learned to praise the team when we did a good job working together. I think I had approximately a week without any issues of getting into the right position. On the last day, I was able to get myself into position quickly. My favorite radiation therapist mumbled "You're perfect." under his breath.

I asked, "What was that, Scott?!" He wasn't going to repeat himself.

I said, "Come on, it's my last day, give me something!"

He raised his voice and said, "You did a good job!"

I like to have silly fun and I don't mind having to do a little flirting along the way, so after the ordeal was all over, I decided that Scott owed me a kiss. He thought I meant I owed *him* a kiss, so he came over to me for a kiss on the cheek. I kissed him then he kissed me on the cheek. We gave each other a kiss on the cheek before a couple of subsequent visits I had at the treatment center. I hope we would if we saw each other today. Being able to have some fun with someone I had spent so much time with during difficult circumstances, made the whole experience worth it! *Finally*, it was over. I left a piece of hot pink duct tape that read, "Good job team!" on one of the boob tubes.

After my last dose of radiation, I went out to the van to see Marcus (who had driven me that day) step out of the vehicle with a half-a-dozen red roses from him and his family! At my request, Mom threw a Radiation Afterglow party so I could celebrate my graduation from radiation with local friends and family the next day. Rather appropriate after that mess...don't you think?

I received a "graduation from radiation" diploma from the radiation team and displayed it proudly at the party! It was fun! The half-a-dozen roses were a beautiful part of the party décor and Tracy's family is still near and dear to my heart.

Lord, thank You for getting us through tough times and allowing us to speak for ourselves. Thank You also for good friends to help us travel through those times. Amen.

~~~

Pick your battles

Cancer is a battle in and of itself. I wish it had been the only battle I had to deal with during treatment, but it was not. Another battle was the bloodwork that I had to have done, usually on a weekly basis.

I have very tiny veins that make having blood drawn difficult. I thought having a port-a-cath would fix all that because it could be used instead of me having to be stuck in a vein each time. Phlebotomists (A.K.A. vampires) must have special training in order to access ports. Having one accessed feels like a needle is being stuck into a piece of soft leather under the skin. I would assume that accessing one also feels different than sticking a needle in a vein for the phlebotomist. I will have to ask one sometime.

For three months, I tried to have bloodwork done through my port with very little success, because the nurses who tried could not get it to return blood, an issue I dealt with earlier in treatment. There were two nurses in the wound care clinic at the hospital who were trained to access ports, but they never had much success with mine either.

The nurse practitioner who was a former cancer nurse had her own ideas about when I needed to do bloodwork and had no qualms about telling my oncologist about this and *rescheduling* my bloodwork for me! As I mentioned before, she was the one who verified that I needed to get my lump checked out and contacted my doctor for me. For that, I am eternally grateful to her. However, it seemed as though her team did not trust that I knew my body as well after the diagnosis just because of the nurse's experience...and that was hard. What was sadly ironic was that the nurse practitioner's husband also had cancer and was seeing the same oncologist I was! She recommended him highly until he became *my* oncologist, as though she lost trust in *him*, too.

Hospitals are as sterile as they can be, but infection can still spread. I had to have a special machine called a "wound vac" that aided in healing hooked up to one of my sores. It had to be changed three times a week by certified nurses, so I had regular appointments in the hospital. My increased time at the hospital came with chronic infections.

When it came time to start chemo, I decided to receive home health care for my pressure sores and later for other personal care, thinking that would decrease my chances of infection. Two of those nurses were able to get the port to work, but due to several unsuccessful attempts prior to that, I decided to ask my surgeon if he wanted my port used when I had my blood drawn.

The surgeon said that he wanted the port to be used for chemo only. Cancer can weaken the immune system, and I was already prone to infection, so it was safer not to use the port unless we had to do so. Oops! I followed his orders until chemo was over. The port worked fine for bloodwork several times after that, and I learned to pick my battles more carefully!

I still caught several infections during treatment. Oh well! You win some...you lose some! I was just glad that those infections never delayed my treatment!

Lord, thank You for helping us pick our battles wisely. Amen.

~~~

Day 25

"It's not the size of the dog in the fight, it's the size of the fight in the dog."
- Mark Twain

Another battle I tried to fight during my journey through treatment had very little to do with my cancer. According to the Department of Revenue Driver's Licensing Board in Topeka, Kansas, I must have medical clearance in order to drive because I have a disability. There is a form that a doctor must fill out annually as an evaluation of my physical, mental and emotional ability to drive, even just to get a learner's permit like most teens do when they go through Drivers Education.

Time to fill out the required form happened to fall as I was starting chemo... but renewing my learner's permit was the *last* thing on my mind. I found out that the company that carried my car insurance would not cover me without a license of some kind, even though I was not the one driving my vehicle at the time. So, I had to do something about it, and *fast!* Getting the form filled out by the primary care doctor I had prior to this was never a problem, but this was a different doctor.

The doctor who called me with my diagnosis was the same one who needed to fill out this form. I have to say she was a very kind, considerate doctor who helped me a lot before this happened. However, having her fill out this simple form was nothing but trouble.

Her office would send me the paperwork and there would be a problem with the way she filled it out (i.e., something missing, she didn't sign it, etc.) After six months of unsuccessfully getting the form filled out – yes - *six months* - I noticed a pattern with something she filled out wrong. I asked the nurse about it. The form asks if the potential driver has any *uncontrolled conditions*. The previous doctor always said *no* because, although I have chronic pressure sores, I *am* in treatment for them often, so he considered them *controlled*. This practitioner didn't see it that way. She put that I had uncontrolled conditions *because* the pressure sores were chronic, and I *was* receiving treatment for them. I talked with the doctor about her response to that one question but couldn't persuade her to change her mind.

If I would have known that it was never going to happen, I wouldn't have tried so hard. There were *so* many other things I could have been doing besides concentrating on that. To top it all off, I was *charged* for having her fill out the form! Eventually, I found a new doctor, and was able to have another one fill out the paperwork correctly, but it still took months.

There were a few other battles I was simply too tired to fight. These battles were exhausting, but I wonder if I would have fought so hard to survive had I not been reminded that I had it in me. At a time when I thought I was "just done" with fighting my battle with cancer, I was reminded by some wonderful people that I *could* keep fighting. The same people reminded me that there were people that could help.

I knew many, many others who had to fight much harder than I did to survive cancer. Some did not survive on Earth for long. Seeing them fight was inspiring.

Lord, thank You for helping us fight our battles. We pray that we fight them using Your will, not ours. Amen.

~~~

<u>Day 26</u>

With God as my Stylist

Since I had heard that radiation can cause hair loss, I told myself I would laugh so hard if my hair started to grow back during radiation. Guess what? It did!

When my hair started to grow back at the beginning of radiation, Mom told me that I looked a little like our friend Sheila. That was such a compliment because Sheila is a beautiful woman with short dark hair with gray *highlights*. As I was explaining to Sheila that I called my hairdo, yep, you guessed it - "*The Sheila*", she thanked me and said she owed her "do" all to her stylist. If I remember correctly, she said his name is Harry. That made me think. Who is *my* stylist?

Having been born with a disability, my body does not always do what I expect it to do. Many times, it does just the opposite. It seldom does everything I would like for it to do. I certainly do not have control over much of what it does.

My hair had been the one constant in my life that I could control. Most of the time I cut it when I wanted to cut it and I let it grow long when I wanted to let it grow long. Cancer changed all that...or maybe God did? The thick, straight hair I was born with came back...thin, curly and unmanageable! I accepted that my hair was going to do whatever it was going to do. God had to style it for me. Yes, I brush my hair, but I found it difficult to do much else with it when it was short and curly.

I wrote "With God as my Stylist" as a devotional to my cancer support group and shared it with Mom. Something in it must have resonated for her, because when I complained about not being able to do anything with my hair she would remind me, "Just be thankful for your Stylist!" I try to remember to be thankful often.

I learned to love the curls. I finally had the "'80's bangs" I had wanted...in the '80's. When God restyled my hair, I started to let Him restyle my life. In some ways I learned to control less, like what other people do with their lives, how they react to me, and certain aspects of my life. In other ways I learned to be in control of more, like my attitude, how I treat others and how I let them treat me.

By the last week of radiation, I did not need to wear my wig. I had been wearing a white cap to treatment, but wore my wig on the last day, just to show it off. God has restyled so much more than my hair in my life. He continues to and will always be my Salvation, my Peacemaker, my Rock and my Redeemer. I need to continue to let Him be my Stylist!

Lord, thank You for being my Stylist. I'm sorry for the times I try to go to a different hairdresser. Amen.

~~~

<u>Day 27</u>

Cancer is not just what you HAVE...it's what you DO.

Long before I *knew* cancer, I knew several people *with* cancer. By watching them I found out that cancer is not just what they *had*...it's what they *did*. Living their lives that way seemed to work for them. When I *met* cancer, I decided to also make it my main focus. Friends and family who had cancer made that look much easier than it was for me.

I have not yet been blessed with a husband or child, so I didn't have to worry about them. I do have a few friends and family members that I check on regularly. Continuing to do so while I had cancer helped me. They were reminders from God that I was not alone and still had purpose.

The biggest struggle I endured was that the rest of my life did not stop while I had cancer. Making cancer a primary focus worked for others. Why not *me*?

I had to put off some tasks I wanted to do (i.e., looking for a job) but still had others that needed done, i.e., laundry, paying bills, etc. There was so much to keep track of and plenty of people reminding me what they thought should be on my "to-do" list. I had to remind some of those people that I needed to take care of my cancer first and foremost. I did find the energy to do an occasional job search, but that was difficult until I knew definitively when treatment would be over.

Fortunately, some of the people who reminded me that so much needed to get done were able to help me check items off my "to-do" list. My apartment lease ran out shortly after I received my diagnosis. I had so many other issues to deal with that even *thinking* about finding another place to live was difficult. Dad helped me with that.

I realized that if I would just ask, I had a lot of help when I needed it. I was grateful to have people that helped me with tasks of daily living every morning and evening, and at times during the day. But, I still yearned to keep my independence.

I was taught to be hyper-vigilant around any nurse, doctor, or attendant care worker because I needed to know what they were doing and if treatment had changed. The home health care nurses did a good job, but that was just one more thing to keep track of and that was exhausting!

At one point I had decided that I had had enough. I admitted to Mom's cousin Teresa that I was completely exhausted and "just done." She reminded me that my parents loved me "more than life itself," and I could reach out to either one of them for help. I felt that love and leaned on them heavily.

My life goes on and it is *beautiful* no matter how hectic. I know people who didn't make cancer what they *did*, just something they *had*, and I admire them for that. I'm glad that worked for them. Having cancer taught me that if I don't let my health be a big focus in my life, I will try not to focus on it at all and pay for it later.

Lord, thank You for helping us through hectic times and reminding us that life is beautiful! Amen.

~~~

Day 28

Survivor 2015

First, I'll tell you more about my survivor shirt. I had my first survivor shirt custom made with a saying from one of the wonderful cards Rachael sent to me. It had a pink ribbon on the top. I love how survivor shirts put the wording in *just* the right place, so the pink ribbon was at the top in the middle. Get the picture? Below the pink ribbon it said,

"Fighter

Fierce

Fantastic"

on the front, and, "I've got a whole different 'F' word for cancer!" in the middle on the back. I wore the lettering off, painted it back on, and wore the shirt so much that it stretched until it was too big. I had a new one made. The lettering is on the front with the word "Fabulous" replacing the word "Fantastic". That was simply a mistake. I guess subconsciously I decided I had a "whole different 'F' word for cancer!" That is a fun way to talk about being a survivor.

The moment I was told I had cancer I felt as though God was telling me I was going to survive it. I had always thought that there was a big, magical moment when one with cancer could say that they were a survivor because they did not have cancer anymore. I have friends that were able to have those moments and I waited for my turn.

I worked so hard! No! I worked *damn* hard to be able to say I was a survivor, but by the time I was, I wondered why I had made such a big deal about it. Believe me, I am grateful that I survived cancer, but the meaning of that word has changed for me.

My attitude toward survival began to change during the final appointment with my radiation oncologist. Usually, we got along great and laughed during my appointments. This one was different. We discussed the fact that I was almost done with treatment. He told me remission is a difficult place to be. Difficult?! What was he talking about?! My cancer support group and I had discussed whether to use the term "remission" or the phrase "I no longer have cancer." When the doctor used the term "remission," I had not yet made the decision to use that word. I know there is always a chance that the cancer will come back, but the way he said "remission" made that possibility sound so absolute.

He and I had the long, gut-wrenching conversation I'm sure he's had with most of his patients. He said that there is no test that says the cancer is no longer there or that it will never come back. Wait! Isn't he the one that told me before radiation that there was no cancer anymore and that radiation was just a preventative measure? Was he confused? I understand that he was speaking from an honest medical standpoint, but that is not what I wanted to hear at the time.

I wanted him to congratulate me and tell me that I had done a good job getting through treatment. I wanted him to tell me chances were slim to none that I would ever have cancer again. What happened was that he talked about the margins which indicate how much good tissue was around the tumor when it was taken out, and the probability of return of the cancer. That's beside the point, because I'm not sure he gave me the correct information about my margins. I honestly thought he was getting my case confused with someone else's. I wanted to get out of there as soon as I could, so I didn't argue with him.

I didn't care if the cancer was going to come back someday. I just wanted to be able to say that I was a survivor, and I wanted to do so now! As the song says, I can go "from zero to sixty in 5.2," at least emotionally, and I did. I burst out crying! Well, this delayed me leaving so soon, but it turned out to be a good thing. He sat down next to me and asked what was wrong. I told him that I wasn't feeling like a survivor. He said he was guessing that at some point in my life I had been told of a certain number of years I could expect to live because of my disability. He was also guessing that I wanted to call myself a survivor because of that. I pictured him waving a magic wand as he said rather flippantly, "So, you're a survivor!" He reminded me I was a survivor because I had survived chemo, radiation, and everything else I have been through in my life. There, *that* was the encouraging, compassionate doctor that I had come to know and love! He said I would feel more like a survivor when the memories of treatment started to fade. I took time to tell him what had been so grueling about radiation, making sure to commend his team of therapists at the end of my spiel.

He shared with me that he had had a long car ride with his wife and three boys that past weekend. I didn't care for his flippant attitude, but I could tell that both of us were exhausted, so I tried to understand. I thanked him for being so kind throughout my treatment. I told him I felt as though he would give me a hug if I asked for one. Our final handshake was a little prolonged because I would not let go until he gave me a hug. Did I mention I'm not afraid to ask for what I want or need?

After that appointment, I began to rethink my ideas about being a survivor. I asked other cancer survivors what they thought about the term. One said she considered herself a survivor because of everything else she had survived in her life...not just the cancer. Another said that "survivor" was a difficult term for her because her mom passed away after having cancer. She had told herself that she was going to wait five years after her diagnosis to begin thinking of herself as a survivor. She can now do so!

Mom and I had a brief discussion about the fact that I could have died. I remember she asked me this question and then answered it for me. "If you had not survived the treatment, would we say you weren't a survivor? No! You have survived a lot in your life!" That conversation turned out to be sadly ironic because Mom and I never talked about the possibility of her death from cancer, just mine. I refuse to think that those who have died of cancer lost, because I know how hard many of them fought.

Some of the memories of my cancer treatment are not as clear as they used to be. Some are still as clear as can be. I'm sure some others will eventually leave me. I don't want them to ever go away completely because they are now part of my story. Maybe I can unload some of them out of my brain once they are published on paper.

Lord, thank You for helping us survive what we go through on Earth so we can ultimately win the war, even if we lose the earthly battle. Amen.

~~~

Day 29

What now?

Another definition I had of the word "survivor" before having cancer was someone that bought a survivor shirt and ran a marathon or had another big accomplishment in his or her life after cancer. I'm still waiting for mine. I think the only marathon I'm running is to and from doctors' appointments! I have many that regularly occur at least twice a year.

I was extremely excited when I finished treatment, and decided it was time to move on with life without cancer. I had an interview in Hutchinson, Kansas the second-to-last week of radiation. Three months later I was offered and accepted the job. I thought this was a way to have a fresh start.

I moved to Junction City, Kansas after I was diagnosed with cancer to be closer to family and friends. Living there made so much sense at a time in life when nothing else did. However, I felt as though I had to move, not just for the job, but for this "new life" in order to get back to the way life was before cancer. I was wrong. It was nice to have a fresh start and as it turned out I would need a new place to call home in the next few years, but life did not go the way I expected after I moved.

Three months after throwing myself into the job, I realized I was no longer taking good care of myself and paying the consequences. The supervisors at my job were not happy with my performance. Truthfully, neither was I.

In that job, I felt as though I was running in a human hamster wheel. You know, those big wheels that you can get into and literally walk in endless circles without going anywhere? Dad pulled my wheelchair into one of those in a park once when I was a little girl. I didn't like it then, and I certainly didn't like being in a job that felt that way. I had worked way too hard to get where I was to feel as though I could never accomplish anything.

After a discussion with my supervisor in which she told me she was not happy with my performance, she made a few suggestions as to how I could improve. This was not the first discussion we had about what she expected from me...but I had a feeling it would be the last. I had already been there for three months and did not see the situation improving.

It did not take long to tell her I did not feel as though I wanted to work that hard to change something I had already been doing for three months. I have learned not to "rat out" my colleagues. I know poor practices will be found out one way or another, but I was a little more honest with her about the way the agency in general was practicing because I thought I could be. After all, I was saying goodbye. What could they do to me?

The day had not started out well. I had a feeling it was going to end the same way. Despite the fact we had had these discussions before, it was easy to take constructive criticism from her because we seemed to be able to reason well. I was grateful she reminded me to pray before I gave her my final answer. I asked her if I could take a break outside. I was the only employee that had access to enter through the back door so I knew if I went out that way I would not be bothered. I said the quickest prayer I have ever prayed. I heard God loudly and clearly tell me to "get out", so I went back in the building to reveal my decision and left the position the next day.

I have not yet found the balance of working outside the home and taking care of myself because that is a full-time job! I have had to take a few years to work solely at the job of taking care of myself. My pressure sores that I had treatment for after chemo and radiation were getting worse because of my long hours at work, and I ended up on bedrest 90% of the time for approximately a year because of it.

Now, don't go feeling sorry for me or thinking I'm lazy...because I am not! Even when I was a kid, I was never good at resting in bed when I was sick. I always had to have something else to do in case I got bored. I am better at resting than I used to be - maybe a little *too* good - but I also keep a bag of activities beside me to occupy my time while I'm in bed. I read a lot. I like to color. During this particular stint of bedrest, I wrote the original rough draft of this book. It took one month.

I should probably rest more often than I do now, but since that long year in bed I have been able to get a battery-operated wheelchair that tilts back to relieve pressure. In fact, recently I got a new one that tilts *and* reclines. Maybe someday we can meet in person and you can see the color! It is called "raspberry beret." French sounding, oui? I call it hot pink...or is it magenta? Anyway, I love it!

I am enjoying being more involved with church activities and more time on my hobbies. I am now a Deacon at church and enjoy helping with our ministry at the local soup kitchen. I am still looking for something major to accomplish. Maybe this book is that accomplishment. Maybe life itself is it.

Life as I know it now has forced me to be a lot less "self-success driven" and a lot more "people-oriented." Maybe surviving cancer for the first time is it. Maybe finding out who I really am and who God intended for me to be is it. Life after cancer is different for everyone. I pray that if you are going through it right now you get to discern what it means for you.

Lord, thank You that there can be life after cancer. Please help us discern who we are in that life. I pray for the loved ones of those who never get to find out. Amen.

~~~

Day 30

"Yeah, I remember him. He stuck a needle in my boob once!"

Okay, as promised, I have shared the complete list of "Things I never thought I'd say." I'm going to explain this one to you. Hopefully, it will give you a good laugh.

There are a couple of procedures that I had to have done before my lumpectomy. I mentioned earlier that I had to have a needle localization prior to my surgery. It is called that, or a needle loc, because a radiologist must put a needle in to guide the surgeon to the area where the lump needs to be removed.

When I had my first post-treatment mammogram I had the help of a technician that I conflicted with during an earlier one. She appeared rude and unaware of how to treat any body, or maybe she was simply unaware of how to treat mine. She was also ignorant of the fact that my battery-operated wheelchair is *mine* and no one is to touch any part of it without my permission. I had my seatbelt on, and she was going to unbuckle it for me! She probably would have moved my wheelchair if I would have let her. When someone else moves my wheelchair without asking I feel as though they are driving while I'm in the driver's seat of my car...and that is *not* okay!

She was much the same way during this mammogram. One of the images taken during the mammogram was not quite good enough and the radiologist, who had also done my needle loc, wanted it retaken so he could look at something more closely. After looking at the second image he came into the room to tell me himself that it was nothing to worry about, just some density.

The technician did not remember me, so I decided to have a little fun with her. She introduced me to the radiologist. I said, "Yeah, I remember him. He stuck a needle in my *boob* once!" I get a kick out of making statements like that just to get a reaction from people! I don't remember her reaction. He acted as though my comment was completely normal and told her that we had just seen each other out in the community.

Lord, thank You again for humor. I pray that I have helped those reading this because I may have experienced something similar to what he or she is going through. Amen.

~~~

Day 31

"No one fights alone." - Brandon Stroda

With his permission I have mentioned my friend Brandon a few times in this book. I have received permission from his wife Terrah to tell you a little more. Their story is important to me.

The quote above was printed on the back of t-shirts worn by hundreds of supporters of Brandon and his family. The t-shirts were printed and sold as a fundraiser to help defray medical expenses during his cancer treatment. The shirts were available in black with white lettering or black and white speckled with white lettering. The black represents melanoma, which is the type of cancer Brandon had for much of his adult life.

"Team Stroda" was a title coined by one of Brandon's doctors when talking to the family about their "village." It is on the front of the shirt. "No one fights alone" is on the back of the shirt and is a phrase Brandon coined himself. He knew he and his family were supported, prayed for, and loved. He has since passed away, but I'm sure he probably knows and delights in the fact that they still are.

Several batches of Team Stroda shirts were made and sold. Someone even made onesies so babies could adorn the attire. Anyone from one month to one-hundred-years-old could wear a shirt, and many did. To say that Team Stroda grew to 1000 members is probably an understatement! Many of us have these t-shirts and wore them on special days during and after his treatment journey. We posted pictures on Facebook of us wearing these shirts. Somebody even started a fun game in which anyone traveling would take the shirt with them and take a picture of them wearing it out of town...or out of the country! The shirts ended up all over the world! Team Stroda still has them and we still wear them occasionally.

I was privileged to be on Brandon's team but even more privileged to have him on mine! He was often the first one in Sunday school to applaud when I mentioned my treatment going well or being done. He always took time to hear what was going on in my life. He was so supportive of anyone going through cancer and other hard times.

His boys are still involved in theater and baseball, two things they loved to do with their dad.

The family supports the community and its members in many ways. Terrah is a great mom and advocate in the community and is also a motivational speaker about their family's journey with Brandon's and her own cancers. She gave me the best pep talk after Mom passed away. I will save the details of that pep talk for my next book.

My team is not nearly as big as Team Stroda, but it is just as important, and I value it greatly! My reason for writing so much about Brandon is to remind you that you are not alone. This book was designed so that I could share my faith, my story, some humor, and to encourage you to do the same when you're ready. I don't mean to steal this phrase from Brandon or his family, but my main goal is to let you know that "no one fights alone."

I am still in this with you. Other readers are in this with you. Your support system is in this with you. Keep going. Fight as hard as you can for as long as you can.

Lord, thank You for our teams. Amen.

~~~

Conclusion

Hello Courage!

I have a picture frame that has muted tones of blues, greens, yellows, a little bit of brown and dark red. Between a pair of butterfly wings at the top is the phrase 'hello courage'. In it is a picture of two people that I think epitomize courage – Grandpa Roy and his great-granddaughter Kylie. I am in the picture looking over my shoulder smiling at them.

Grandpa Roy is in his nineties and is still setting life goals. He bought a motorcycle when he was eighty. It was neither his first nor his last! When he was eighty-nine, he decided to learn to play bridge. He set another goal when he turned ninety. And another when he was ninety-one. And...you get the idea. When he turned ninety-three, I asked him what his goal was for the year. He told me then that he wasn't sure what he had left to do. He is ninety-four-years-old and found out last year that he was a good candidate for a pacemaker. He and his doctor pursued this idea, while examining other possible reasons for his low energy. He had the surgery because he wanted more energy than he has had in a while! The surgery came with some ups and downs, but he is still surviving!

Kylie is a fearless eight-year-old. In my opinion, it goes without saying that she is courageous because she is a child. Like many other children in my family who are fearless at a young age, she used to climb up anything and jump off with the courage and faith of a child who knew someone was always going to catch her.

Her mom Jenni and I discussed Kylie's courage once. Jenni said that Kylie still has a lot of courage and gave the example of the intruder drills they have at her school now. Although it is sad, they have drills to teach the kids what to do in case a shooter or some other bad person comes into the school. Jenni was there during one of these drills and said that Kylie handled it as though it was part of a normal school day!

I know many people who have a lot of courage. However, I have trouble when that word is spoken about me. When people tell me that I've had a lot of courage to get through everything I've been through in life, I just think, "That wasn't courage! That was survival!"

In her TED Talk "The Power of Vulnerability", Brené Brown explains that courage comes from the Latin word "cor" which means "heart." The first definition of it when it was brought into the English language was "to tell the story of who you are with your whole heart."[3] Her TED talks are amazing! I highly recommend them.

---

[3] **TED.** (2010, June), Brené Brown: The Power of Vulnerability {Video File} Retrieved from
htttps://www.ted.com/talks/brene_brown_on_vulnerability?language =en.

I've written my story as raw, real, honest and whole-hearted as I know how. So, if you want to say that I have courage because I wrote this book, I'll take it, and thank you! I pray that you have the courage to write, or at least tell your story whenever you are ready.

This may not be the end of the journey, but it is the end of this book. I hope you enjoyed it! My thoughts and my life have changed a lot since I began to write this book. A few of my current thoughts have snuck their way in!

This is not designed to be a "do this, not that" or "this is exactly what cancer is like" sort of book. As my friend Ron would probably say, I'm just giving you the "Clif Notes" of my experience with cancer treatment. The Clif Notes are rather detailed, I know. You're welcome.

After Mom's Celebration of Life service, a friend sat down next to me and said, "Now you have another book to write." Without even thinking, I said, "Yes, I do." I am strongly considering it! We'll see how this one goes.

While going through cancer I decided I needed a life mantra. At first mine was, "Today's a new day!" I decided that saying that throughout the day didn't make much sense, so, then the mantra was, "Tomorrow's a new day!" I used that for a while. I'm sure I had more than one grueling day when I stated, "Tomorrow's another day!" I didn't always mean that one positively. I decided on the last day of treatment that, "*Life is beautiful*!" I still use that mantra to this day. So, as you are waiting to see if, and when, I write again, remember that *life is beautiful!*

References

1. Gaither, G. and Gaither, W. (1971) Because He Lives

2. Lynn, R. L. (2013) Cancer is so Limited and Other Poems of Faith. United States. CreateSpace

3. **TED.** (2010, June). Brené Brown: The Power of Vulnerability [Video file] Retrieved from https://www.ted.com/talks/brené_brown_on_vulnerability?language=en.

About the Author

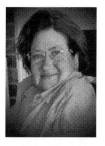

Hi! I'm Melody J. Cole. Thank you for meeting me here! In the past, I was blessed with many opportunities to co-author and/or present on various topics. This is my first solo writing project that I have self-published. My hope is that you are reading this by the time I celebrate my fifth anniversary of surviving breast cancer - July 2, 2020.

Currently, I enjoy life in South Hutchinson, Kansas with my fur teen Earl of Whiskers. I love spending time with friends and family. I am a member and Deacon of First Presbyterian Church of Hutchinson, Kansas.

I strive to use my God-given creativity wisely through writing, public speaking and art. Please come visit my Sentiments of a Survivor page on Facebook for exciting happenings with the book, to "have the conversation" by private Facebook message, and to learn a bit more about me. I would love to meet you!

Made in the USA
Middletown, DE
27 September 2020

20649739R00057